A Beginners Guide to Plant Based Diet Recipes

Start Cooking with Easy Recipes for Eat Healthy
Foods and Lose Weight without Sacrificing
Taste.

Valerie Harvey

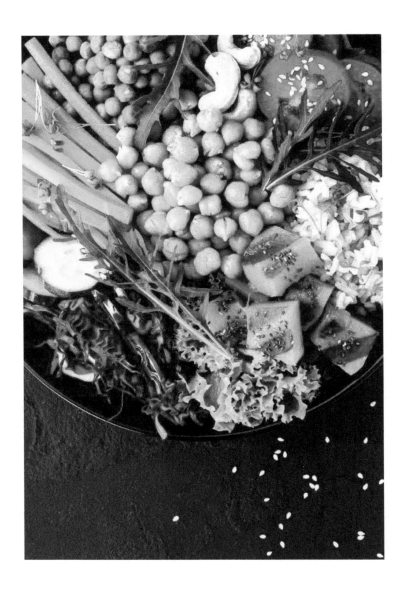

Table of Contents

The information in the following pages is broadly considered a truthful and accurate account of facts and as such, any inattention, use, or misuse of the information in question by the reader will render any resulting actions solely under their purview. There are no scenarios in which the publisher or the original author of this work can be in any fashion deemed liable for any hardship or damages that may befall them after undertaking information described herein.

Additionally, the information in the following pages is intended only for informational purposes and should thus be thought of as universal. As befitting its nature, it is presented without assurance regarding its prolonged validity or interim quality. Trademarks that are mentioned are done without written consent and can in no way be considered an endorsement from the trademark holder.

Introduction

A plant-based diet is a diet based primarily on whole plant foods. It is identical to the regular diet we're used to already, except that it leaves out foods that are not exclusively from plants. Hence, a plant-based diet does away with all types of animal-sourced foods, hydrogenated oils, refined sugars, and processed foods. A whole food plant-based diet comprises not just fruits and vegetables; it also consists of unprocessed or barely-processed oils with healthy monounsaturated fats (like extra-virgin olive oil), whole grains, legumes (essentially lentils and beans), seeds and nuts, as well as herbs and spices.

What makes a plant-based meal (or any meal) fun is the manner with which you make them; the seasoning process; and the combination process that contributes to a fantastic flavor and makes every meal unique and enjoyable. There are lots of delicious recipes (all plant-centered), which will prove helpful in when you intend making mouthwatering, healthy plant-based dishes for personal or household consumption. Provided you're eating these plant-based foods regularly, you'll have very problems with fat or diseases that result from bad dietary habits, and there would be no need for excessive calorie tracking.

Plant-based diet recipes are versatile; they range from colorful Salads to Lentil Stews, and Bean Burritos. The recipes also draw influences from around the globe, with Mexican, Chinese, European, Indian cuisines all part of the vast array of plant-based recipes available to choose from. Why You Ought to Reduce Your Intake of Processed and Animal-Based Foods. You have likely heard over and over that processed food has adverse effects on your health. You might have also been told repeatedly to stay away from foods with lots of preservatives; nevertheless, nobody ever offered any genuine or concrete facts about why you ought to avoid these foods and why they are unsafe. Consequently, let us properly dissect it to help you properly comprehend why you ought to stay away from these healthy eating offenders. They have massive habit-forming characteristics. Humans have a predisposition towards being addicted to some specific foods; however, the reality is that the fault is not wholly ours. Every one of the unhealthy treats we relish now and then triggers the dopamine release in our brains. This creates a pleasurable effect in our brain, but the excitement is usually short-lived. The discharged dopamine additionally causes an attachment connection gradually, and this is the reason some people consistently go back to eat certain unhealthy foods even when they know it's unhealthy and unnecessary. You can get rid of this by taking out that inducement completely. They are sugar-laden and plenteous in glucose-fructose syrup. Animal-based and processed foods are laden with refined sugars and glucose-fructose syrup which has almost no beneficial food nutrient. An ever-increasing number of studies are affirming what several people presumed from the start; that genetically modified foods bring about inflammatory bowel disease, which consequently makes it increasingly difficult for the body to assimilate essential nutrients. The disadvantages that result from your body being unable to assimilate essential nutrients from consumed foods rightly cannot be overemphasized. Processed and animal-based food products contain plenteous amounts of refined carbohydrates. Indeed, your body requires carbohydrates to give it the needed energy to run body capacities. In any case, refining carbs dispenses with the fundamental supplements; in the way that refining entire grains disposes of the whole grain part. What remains, in the wake of refining, is what's considered as empty carbs or empty calories. These can negatively affect the metabolic system in your body by sharply increasing your blood sugar and insulin quantities. They contain lots of synthetic

—

ingredients. At the point when your body is taking in non-natural ingredients, it regards them as foreign substances. Your body treats them as a health threat. Your body isn't accustomed to identifying synthetic compounds like sucralose or these synthesized sugars. Hence, in defense of your health against this foreign "aggressor," your body does what it's capable of to safeguard your health. It sets off an immune reaction to tackle this "enemy" compound, which indirectly weakens your body's general disease alertness, making you susceptible to illnesses. The concentration and energy expended by your body in ensuring your immune system remain safe could instead be devoted somewhere else. They contain constituent elements that set off an excitable reward sensation in your body. A part of processed and animal-based foods contain compounds like glucose-fructose syrup, monosodium glutamate, and specific food dyes that can trigger some addiction. They rouse your body to receive a benefit in return whenever you consume them. Monosodium glutamate, for example, is added to many store-bought baked foods. This additive slowly conditions your palates to relish the taste. It gets mental just by how your brain interrelates with your taste sensors.

This reward-centric arrangement makes you crave it increasingly, which ends up exposing you to the danger of over consuming calories.

For animal protein, usually, the expression "subpar" is used to allude to plant proteins since they generally have lower levels of essential amino acids as against animal-sourced protein. Nevertheless, what the vast majority don't know is that large amounts of essential amino acids can prove detrimental to your health. Let me break it down further for you.

Mediterranean Veggie Wrap

Preparation time: 15 Minutes
Cooking time: 0 Minutes
Servings: 4
Ingredients:

- Whole-grain Tortillas (
- Chickpeas (3 C.)
- Onion (1/4 C., Diced)
- Tomato (1, Diced)
- Salt (to Taste)
- Kalamata Olives (4 T.)
- Garlic Clove (1, Minced)
- Lettuce (2 C.)
- Lemon Juice (2 T.)
- Cucumber (1, Grated)
- Fresh Dill (2 T.)
- Plant-based Yogurt (7 Oz.)
- Green Pepper (1/4 C., Diced)

- Pepper (to Taste)

Directions:

1. Before you begin preparing this wrap, you will want to take half of your cucumber and grate it into a mixing bowl.

2. After this step is complete, lightly sprinkle the cucumber with salt to help get some of the excess water out.

3. As this process happens, you can now take your chickpeas and mash them down well with a fork.

4. With that, all set, take out a dish, and combine the cucumber, yogurt, citrus juice, garlic, and dill altogether. Once this is done, season with pepper and salt to your liking.

5. When you are ready, lay out your wraps and layer your smashed chickpeas, lettuce, and the mixed vegetables. For some extra flavor, try adding some tzatziki sauce over the top before rolling up.

Nutrition:

Calories: 400, Carbs: 30g, Fats: 5g

Proteins: 15g

Quick Lentil Wrap

Preparation time: 10 Minutes

Cooking time: 30 Minutes

Servings: 4

Ingredients:

- Whole-grain Wraps (

- Garlic Clove (1, Minced)

- Olive Oil (2 T.)

- Onion (1, Diced)

- Cilantro (1/3 C., Cilantro)

- Lentils (2 C.)

- Tomato Paste (1/3 C.)

Directions:

1. Begin this recipe by taking out a skillet and place two cups of water and lentils in.

2. You will want to get everything to a boil before turning the temperature down and simmer for ten minutes or until the lentils are soft.

3. Once the lentils are cooked through, add in the tomato paste, garlic, and onion. Go ahead and cook all of these **Ingredients:** together for another five minutes before turning off heat and seasoning to your liking.

4. Finally, lay out your wraps, spread the mixture in the center, and then roll the wrap up for lunch.

Nutrition:

Calories: 400

Carbs: 50g

Fats: 5g

Proteins: 20g

Thai Vegetable and Tofu Wrap

Preparation time: 5 Minutes

Cooking time: 30 Minutes

Servings: 1

Ingredients:

- Extra-firm Tofu (1 C., Diced)

- Peanut Sauce (1/4 C.)

- Olive Oil (1 t.)

- Cucumber (1/3 C., Diced)

- Carrot (1/3 C., Shredded)

- Cilantro (1/4 C.)

- Garlic Cloves (1, Minced)

- Whole-wheat Wrap (

Directions:

1. Tofu is an excellent Protein to have on hand because it is so versatile! To begin this recipe, you will want to take a skillet and place it over medium heat.

2. As it warms, add in your olive oil and begin cooking the tofu for around five minutes.

3. After five minutes, combine in the garlic and cook for an additional minute. At this point, all of the liquid from the tofu should be gone.

4. Next, eliminate the skillet from the cooker and add in the peanut sauce. Be sure to stir very well to help coat the tofu pieces evenly!

5. When you are set to make your wraps, spread the tofu into your wrap, top with the diced and shredded vegetables, and roll everything up together nice and tight before serving.

6. For extra flavor, feel free to add some fresh cilantro to your wrap!

Nutrition:

Calories: 270

Carbs: 12g

Fats: 15g

Proteins: 20g

Plant-based Buffalo Wrap

Preparation time: 5 Minutes

Cooking time: 15 Minutes

Servings: 4

Ingredients:

- Olive Oil (1 t.)

- Kale (2 C., Chopped)

- Buffalo Sauce (1/2 C.)

- Seitan (1 C., Chopped)

- Whole Wheat Wraps (

- Tomatoes (1 C., Diced)

- Cashews (1 C.)

- Salt (to taste)

- Dried Dill (1/2 t.)

- Pepper (to Taste)

- Dried Parsley (1/2 t.)

- Almond Milk (8 T.)

- Apple Cider Vinegar (1 ½ T.)

Directions:

1. You can accomplish this by taking out your blender and mixing together the almond milk, apple cider vinegar, cashews, pepper, salt, parsley, and dill together.

2. Once this is done, set your sauce to the side.

3. Next, you will need to get out a saucepan and place it over medium heat. Once warm, add in some olive oil and begin cooking your seitan pieces. Normally, this will take you eight minutes.

4. When the seitan is cooked through, add in the buffalo sauce and cook for another minute.

5. With these steps done, you will want to now take a moment to take the kale and mix it in a bowl with olive oil and seasoning.

6. Finally, it is time to assemble your wrap! You can do this by taking out your wrap and spreading your ranch dressing across the surface.

7. Once this is in place, begin building your wrap by layering the kale, tomato, and seitan pieces. For a final touch, add some more buffalo sauce over the top and then wrap it up!

Nutrition:

Calories: 250

Carbs: 25g

Fats: 15g

Proteins: 20g

Colorful Veggie Wrap

Preparation time: 10 Minutes

Cooking time: 0 Minutes

Servings: 4

Ingredients:

- Large Lettuce Leaves (

- Soy Sauce (1 T.)

- Olive Oil (1 T.)

- Seed Butter (1/2 C.)

- Garlic Powder (1 T.)

- Lime Juice (2 T.)

- Red Cabbage (1 C., Shredded)

- Cucumber (1 C., Chopped)

- Red Pepper (1 C., Chopped)

- Carrot (1 C., Chopped)

- Ground Ginger (1/4 t.)

Directions:

1. This wrap looks pretty at and full of flavor! You can start this recipe off by making the sauce.

2. For the sauce, take out a petite bowl and combine together the oil, garlic, soy sauce, juice of the lime, ground ginger, pepper flakes, and the seed butter.

3. Once everything is mixed together well, place it to the side.

4. Next, it is time to build your wrap! Go ahead and lay the lettuce leaves out flat before spreading sauce across the surface.

5. Once this is in place, you will want to layer the other vegetables before rolling the leaf up and enjoying your veggie-packed wrap!

Nutrition:

Calories: 250

Carbs: 15g

Fats: 20g

Proteins: 10g

BBQ Chickpea Wrap

Preparation time: 10 Minutes

Cooking time: 0 Minutes

Servings: 4

Ingredients:

- Whole-wheat Tortillas (

- Coleslaw (2 C.)

- BBQ Sauce (1/2 C.)

- Chickpeas (2 C.)

Directions:

1. Are you in a rush for lunch? You can slap this wrap together in a snap! Start off by taking out a blending bowl and combine the BBQ with the chickpeas.

2. Next, you will want to lay out your tortillas and place the coleslaw and chickpeas in the center.

3. For a nice touch, wrap your tortilla up and pop into the microwave for a few seconds to heat it up before enjoying it!

Nutrition:

Calories: 450, Carbs: 50g, Fats: 5g, Proteins: 10g

Chickpea and Mango Wraps

Preparation time: 15 minutes

Cooking time: 0 minutes

Servings: 3

Ingredients:

- 3 tablespoons tahini

- 1 tablespoon curry powder

- ¼ teaspoon sea salt (optional)

- Zest and juice of 1 lime

- 3 to 4 tablespoons water

- 1½ cups cooked chickpeas

- 1 cup diced mango

- ½ cup fresh cilantro, chopped

- 1 red bell pepper, deseeded and diced

- 3 large whole-wheat wraps

- 1½ cups shredded lettuce

Directions:

1. In a large bowl, stir together the tahini, curry powder, lime zest, lime juice and sea salt (if desired) until smooth and creamy. Whisk in 3 to 4 tablespoons water to help thin the mixture.

2. Add the cooked chickpeas, mango, cilantro and bell pepper to the bowl. Toss until well coated.

3. On a clean work surface, lay the wraps. Divide the chickpea and mango mixture among the wraps. Spread the shredded lettuce on top and roll up tightly.

4. Serve immediately.

Nutrition:

Calories: 436

Fat: 17.9g

Carbs: 8.9g

Protein: 15.2g

Fiber: 12.1g

Tofu and Pineapple in Lettuce

Preparation time: 2 hours

Cooking time: 15 minutes

Servings: 4

Ingredients:

- ¼ cup low-sodium soy sauce

- 1 garlic clove, minced

- 2 tablespoons sesame oil (optional)

- 1 tablespoons coconut sugar (optional)

- 1 (14-ounce / 397-g) package extra firm tofu, drained, cut into ½-inch cubes

- 1 small white onion, diced

- ½ pineapple, peeled, cored, cut into cubes

- Salt and ground black pepper, to taste (optional)

- 4 large lettuce leaves

- 1 tablespoon roasted sesame seeds

Directions:

1. Combine the soy sauce, garlic, sesame oil (if desired), and coconut sugar in a bowl. Stir to mix well.

2. Add the tofu cubes to the bowl of soy sauce mixture, then press to coat well. Wrap the bowl in plastic and refrigerate to marinate for at least 2 hours.

3. Pour the marinated tofu and marinade in a skillet and heat over medium heat. Add the onion and pineapple cubes to the skillet and stir to mix well.

4. Sprinkle with salt (if desired) and pepper and sauté for 15 minutes or until the onions are lightly browned and the pineapple cubes are tender.

5. Divide the lettuce leaves among 4 plates, then top the leaves with the tofu and pineapple mixture. Sprinkle with sesame seeds and serve immediately.

Nutrition:

Calories: 259

Fat: 15.4g

Carbs: 20.5g

Protein: 12.1g

Fiber: 3.2g

Quinoa and Black Bean Lettuce Wraps

Preparation time: 30 minutes

Cooking time: 15 minutes

Servings: 6

Ingredients:

- 2 tablespoons avocado oil (optional)

- ¼ cup deseeded and chopped bell pepper

- ½ onion, chopped

- 2 tablespoons minced garlic

- 1 teaspoon salt (optional)

- 1 teaspoon pepper (optional)

- ½ cup cooked quinoa

- 1 cup cooked black beans

- ½ cup almond flour

- ½ teaspoon paprika

- ½ teaspoon red pepper flakes

- 6 large lettuce leaves

Directions:

1. Heat 1 tablespoon of the avocado oil (if desired) in a skillet over medium-high heat.

2. Add the bell peppers, onions, garlic, salt (if desired), and pepper. Sauté for 5 minutes or until the bell peppers are tender.

3. Turn off the heat and allow to cool for 10 minutes, then pour the vegetables in a food processor. Add the quinoa, beans, flour.

4. Sprinkle with paprika and red pepper flakes. Pulse until thick and well combined.

5. Line a baking pan with parchment paper, then shape the mixture into 6 patties with your hands and place on the baking pan.

6. Put the pan in the freezer for 5 minutes to make the patties firm.

7. Heat the remaining avocado oil (if desired) in the skillet over high heat.

8. Add the patties and cook for 6 minutes or until well browned on both sides. Flip the patties halfway through.

9. Arrange the patties in the lettuce leaves and serve immediately.

Nutrition:

Calories: 200

Fat: 10.6g

Carbs: 40.5g

Protein: 9.5g

Fiber: 8.2g

Smoothies and Beverages

Kale Smoothie

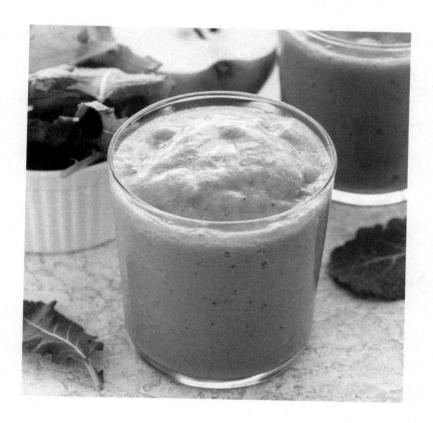

Preparation Time: 5 minutes

Cooking Time: 0 minutes

Servings: 2

Ingredients:

- 2 cups chopped kale leaves
- 1 banana, peeled
- 1 cup frozen strawberries
- 1 cup unsweetened almond milk
- 4 Medjool dates, pitted and chopped

Directions:

1. Put all the ingredients in a food processor, then blitz until glossy and smooth.
2. Serve immediately or chill in the refrigerator for an hour before serving.

Nutrition:

Calories: 663

Fat: 10.0g

Carbs: 142.5g

Fiber: 19.0g

Protein: 17.4g

Hot Tropical Smoothie

Preparation Time: 5 minutes

Cooking Time: 0 minutes

Servings: 4

Ingredients:

- 1 cup frozen mango chunks
- 1 cup frozen pineapple chunks
- 1 small tangerine, peeled and pitted
- 2 cups spinach leaves
- 1 cup coconut water
- ¼ teaspoon cayenne pepper, optional

Directions:

1. Add all the ingredients in a food processor, then blitz until the mixture is smooth and combine well.
2. Serve immediately or chill in the refrigerator for an hour before serving.

Nutrition:

Calories: 283,Fat: 1.9g,Carbs: 67.9g,Fiber: 10.4g, Protein: 6.4g

Berry Smoothie

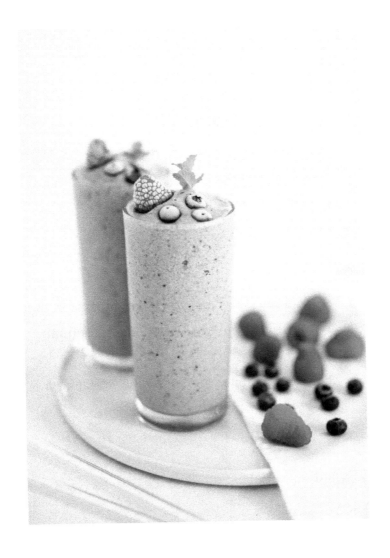

Preparation Time: 5 minutes

Cooking Time: 0 minutes

Servings: 4

Ingredients:

1 cup berry mix (strawberries, blueberries, and cranberries)
4 Medjool dates, pitted and chopped
1½ cups unsweetened almond milk, plus more as needed

Directions:

Add all the ingredients in a blender, then process until the mixture is smooth and well mixed.
Serve immediately or chill in the refrigerator for an hour before serving.

Nutrition:

Calories: 473

Fat: 4.0g

Carbs: 103.7g

Fiber: 9.7g

Protein: 14.8g

Cranberry and Banana Smoothie

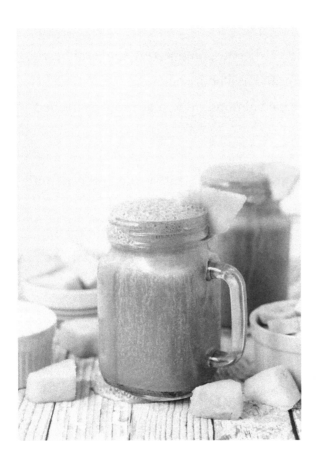

Preparation Time: 5 minutes

Cooking Time: 0 minutes

Servings: 4

1 cup frozen cranberries

1 large banana, peeled

4 Medjool dates, pitted and chopped

1½ cups unsweetened almond milk

Directions:

Add all the ingredients in a food processor, then process until the mixture is glossy and well mixed. Serve immediately or chill in the refrigerator for an hour before serving.

Nutrition:

Calories: 616

Fat: 8.0g

Carbs: 132.8g

Fiber: 14.6g

Protein: 15.7g

Pumpkin Smoothie

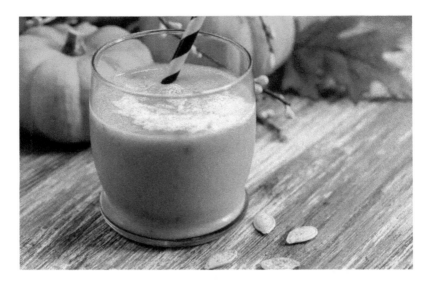

Preparation Time: 5 minutes

Cooking Time: 0 minutes

Servings: 5

Ingredients:

½ cup pumpkin purée

4 Medjool dates, pitted and chopped

1 cup unsweetened almond milk

¼ teaspoon vanilla extract

¼ teaspoon ground cinnamon

½ cup ice

Pinch ground nutmeg

Directions:

Add all the ingredients in a blender, then process until the mixture is glossy and well mixed.
Serve immediately.

Nutrition:

Calories: 417

Fat: 3.0g

Carbs: 94.9g

Fiber: 10.4g

Protein: 11.4g

Super Smoothie

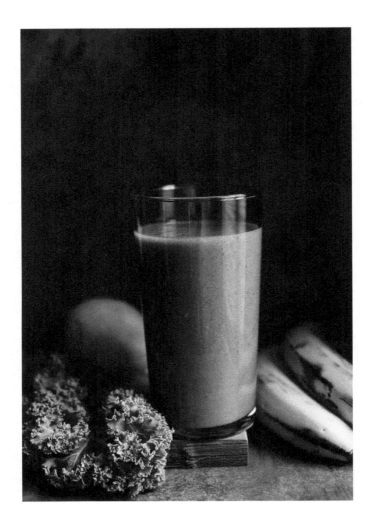

Preparation Time: 5 minutes

Cooking Time: 0 minutes

Servings: 4

Ingredients:

1 banana, peeled

1 cup chopped mango

1 cup raspberries

¼ cup rolled oats

1 carrot, peeled

1 cup chopped fresh kale

2 tablespoons chopped fresh parsley

1 tablespoon flaxseeds

1 tablespoon grated fresh ginger

½ cup unsweetened soy milk

1 cup water

Directions:

Put all the ingredients in a food processor, then blitz
until glossy and smooth.

Serve immediately or chill in the refrigerator for an
hour before serving.

Nutrition:

Calories: 550

Fat: 39.0g

Carbs: 31.0g

Fiber: 15.0g

Protein: 13.0g

Kiwi and Strawberry Smoothie

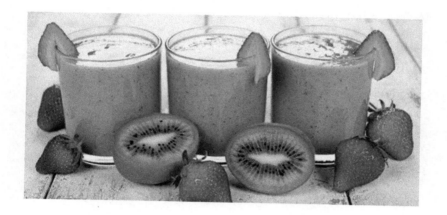

Preparation Time: 5 minutes

Cooking Time: 0 minutes

Servings: 3

Ingredients:

1 kiwi, peeled

5 medium strawberries

½ frozen banana

1 cup unsweetened almond milk

2 tablespoons hemp seeds

2 tablespoons peanut butter

1 to 2 teaspoons maple syrup

½ cup spinach leaves

Handful broccoli sprouts

Directions:

Put all the ingredients in a food processor, then blitz
until creamy and smooth.

Serve immediately or chill in the refrigerator for an
hour before serving.

Nutrition:

Calories: 562

Fat: 28.6g

Carbs: 63.6g

Fiber: 15.1g

Protein: 23.3g

Banana and Chai Chia Smoothie

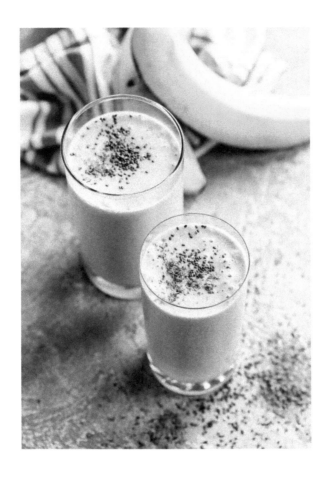

Preparation Time: 5 minutes

Cooking Time: 0 minutes

Servings: 3

Ingredients:

1 banana

1 cup alfalfa sprouts

1 tablespoon chia seeds

½ cup unsweetened coconut milk

1 to 2 soft Medjool dates, pitted

¼ teaspoon ground cinnamon

1 tablespoon grated fresh ginger

1 cup water

Pinch ground cardamom

Directions:

Add all the ingredients in a blender, then process until the mixture is smooth and creamy. Add water or coconut milk if necessary.

Serve immediately.

Nutrition:

Calories: 477,Fat: 41.0g,Carbs: 31.0g,Fiber: 14.0g,Protein: 8.0g

Chocolate and Peanut Butter Smoothie

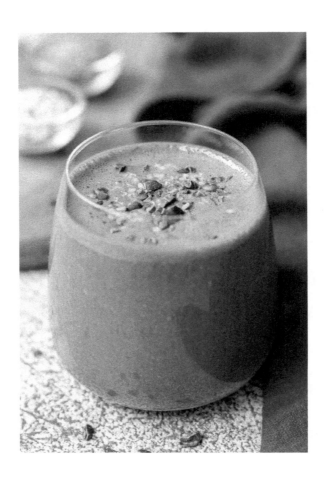

Preparation Time: 5 minutes

Cooking Time: 0 minutes

Servings: 4

Ingredients:

- 1 tablespoon unsweetened cocoa powder
- 1 tablespoon peanut butter
- 1 banana
- 1 teaspoon maca powder
- ½ cup unsweetened soy milk
- ¼ cup rolled oats
- 1 tablespoon flaxseeds
- 1 tablespoon maple syrup
- 1 cup water

Directions:

Add all the ingredients in a blender, then process until the mixture is smooth and creamy. Add water or soy milk if necessary.

Serve immediately.

Nutrition:

Calories: 474

Fat: 16.0g

Carbs: 27.0g

Fiber: 18.0g

Protein: 13.0g

Golden Milk

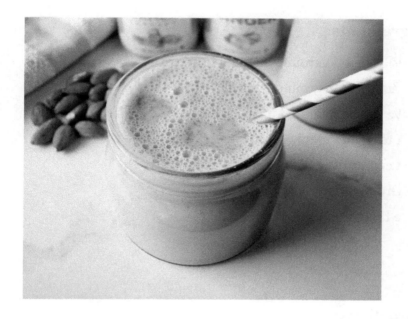

Preparation Time: 5 minutes

Cooking Time: 0 minutes

Servings: 4

Ingredients:

¼ teaspoon ground cinnamon

½ teaspoon ground turmeric

½ teaspoon grated fresh ginger

1 teaspoon maple syrup

1 cup unsweetened coconut milk

Ground black pepper, to taste

2 tablespoon water

Directions:

Combine all the ingredients in a saucepan. Stir to mix well.

Heat over medium heat for 5 minutes. Keep stirring during the heating.

Allow to cool for 5 minutes, then pour the mixture in a blender. Pulse until creamy and smooth. Serve immediately.

Nutrition:

Calories: 577

Fat: 57.3g

Carbs: 19.7g

Fiber: 6.1g

Protein: 5.7g

Mango Agua Fresca

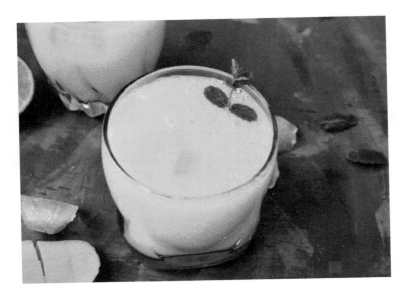

Preparation Time: 5 minutes

Cooking Time: 0 minutes

Servings: 2

Ingredients:

 2 fresh mangoes, diced

 1½ cups water

 1 teaspoon fresh lime juice

 Maple syrup, to taste

 2 cups ice

 2 slices fresh lime, for garnish

 2 fresh mint sprigs, for garnish

Directions:

Put the mangoes, lime juice, maple syrup, and water in
a blender. Process until creamy and smooth.
Divide the beverage into two glasses, then garnish each
glass with ice, lime slice, and mint sprig before
serving.

Nutrition:

Calories: 230

Fat: 1.3g

Carbs: 57.7g

Fiber: 5.4g

Protein: 2.8g

Light Ginger Tea

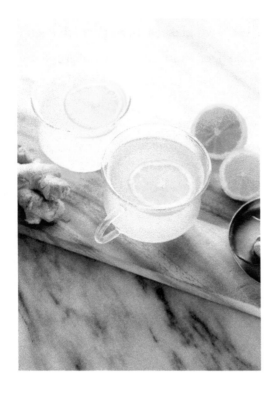

Preparation Time: 5 minutes

Cooking Time: 10 to 15 minutes

Servings: 2

Ingredients:

1 small ginger knob, sliced into four 1-inch chunks

4 cups water

Juice of 1 large lemon

Maple syrup, to taste

Directions:

Add the ginger knob and water in a saucepan, then simmer over medium heat for 10 to 15 minutes. Turn off the heat, then mix in the lemon juice. Strain the liquid to remove the ginger, then fold in the maple syrup and serve.

Nutrition:

Calories: 32

Fat: 0.1g

Carbs: 8.6g

Fiber: 0.1g

Protein: 0.1g

Classic Switchel

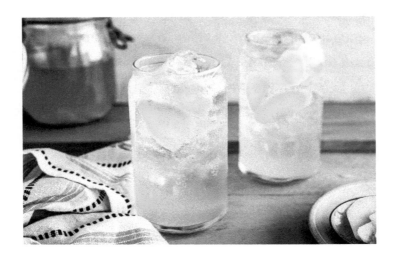

Preparation Time: 5 minutes

Cooking Time: 0 minutes

Servings: 4

Ingredients:

- 1-inch piece ginger, minced
- 2 tablespoons apple cider vinegar
- 2 tablespoons maple syrup
- 4 cups water
- ¼ teaspoon sea salt, optional

Directions:

Combine all the ingredients in a glass. Stir to mix well. Serve immediately or chill in the refrigerator for an hour before serving.

Nutrition:

Calories: 110

Fat: 0g

Carbs: 28.0g

Fiber: 0g

Protein: 0g

Lime and Cucumber Electrolyte Drink

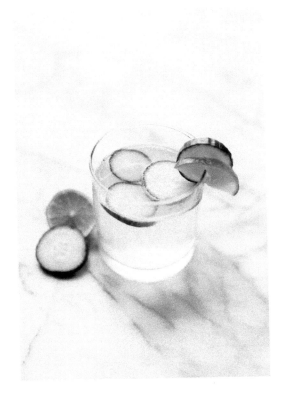

Preparation Time: 5 minutes

Cooking Time: 0 minutes

Servings: 4

Ingredients:

¼ cup chopped cucumber

1 tablespoon fresh lime juice

1 tablespoon apple cider vinegar

2 tablespoons maple syrup

¼ teaspoon sea salt, optional

4 cups water

Directions:

Combine all the ingredients in a glass. Stir to mix well. Refrigerate overnight before serving.

Nutrition:

Calories: 114

Fat: 0.1g

Carbs: 28.9g

Fiber: 0.3g

Protein: 0.3g

Easy and Fresh Mango Madness

Preparation Time: 5 minutes

Cooking Time: 0 minutes

Servings: 4

Ingredients:

- 1 cup chopped mango
- 1 cup chopped peach
- 1 banana
- 1 cup strawberries
- 1 carrot, peeled and chopped
- 1 cup water

Directions:

Put all the ingredients in a food processor, then blitz until glossy and smooth.

Serve immediately or chill in the refrigerator for an hour before serving.

Nutrition:

Calories: 376

Fat: 22.0g

Carbs: 19.0g

Fiber: 14.0g

Protein: 5.0g

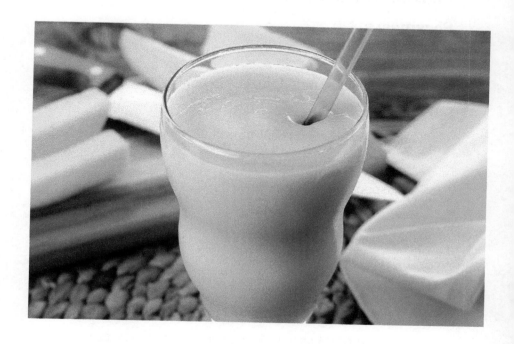

Simple Date Shake

Preparation Time: 10 minutes

Cooking Time: 0 minutes

Servings: 2

Ingredients:

  5 Medjool dates, pitted, soaked in boiling water for 5
    minutes

  ¾ cup unsweetened coconut milk

  1 teaspoon vanilla extract

  ½ teaspoon fresh lemon juice

  ¼ teaspoon sea salt, optional

  1½ cups ice

Directions:

  Put all the ingredients in a food processor, then blitz
    until it has a milkshake and smooth texture.
  Serve immediately.

Nutrition:

Calories: 380

Fat: 21.6g

Carbs: 50.3g

Fiber: 6.0g

Protein: 3.2g

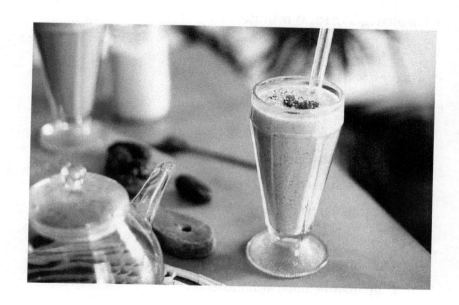

Beet and Clementine Protein Smoothie

Preparation Time: 10 minutes

Cooking Time: 0 minutes

Servings: 3

Ingredients:

- 1 small beet, peeled and chopped
- 1 clementine, peeled and broken into segments
- ½ ripe banana
- ½ cup raspberries
- 1 tablespoon chia seeds
- 2 tablespoons almond butter
- ¼ teaspoon vanilla extract
- 1 cup unsweetened almond milk
- 1/8 teaspoon fine sea salt, optional

Directions:

Combine all the ingredients in a food processor, then pulse on high for 2 minutes or until glossy and creamy.

Refrigerate for an hour and serve chilled.

Nutrition:

Calories: 526

Fat: 25.4g

Carbs: 61.9g

Fiber: 17.3g

Protein: 20.6g

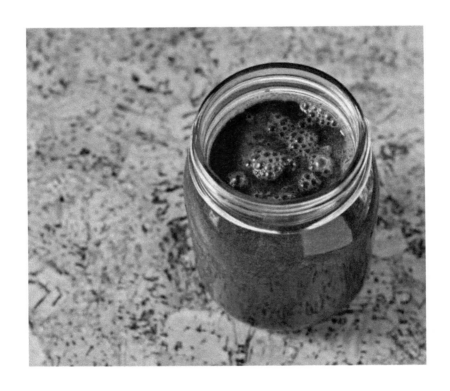

Matcha Limeade

Preparation Time: 10 minutes

Cooking Time: 0 minutes

Servings: 4

Ingredients:

2 tablespoons matcha powder

¼ cup raw agave syrup

3 cups water, divided

1 cup fresh lime juice

3 tablespoons chia seeds

Directions:

Lightly simmer the matcha, agave syrup, and 1 cup of water in a saucepan over medium heat. Keep stirring until no matcha lumps.

Pour the matcha mixture in a large glass, then add the remaining ingredients and stir to mix well.

Refrigerate for at least an hour before serving.

Nutrition:

Calories: 152

Fat: 4.5g

Carbs: 26.8g

Fiber: 5.3g

Protein: 3.7g

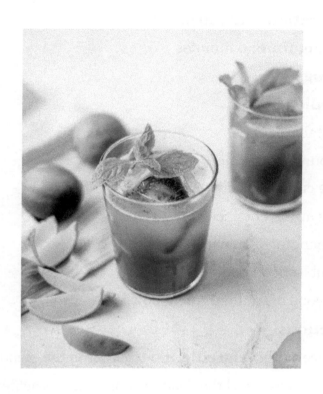

Green & Mean

Preparation time: 10 minutes

Cooking time: 0 minutes

Servings: 1

Ingredients:

3 stalks of Celery

3 bunches of Kale

1/2 cup of sliced pineapple

1/2 apple, chopped

A handful of spinach

1 tablespoon of coconut oil

1 scoop of vanilla Protein powder

Directions:

Place all the **Ingredients:** together in the blender and process until the desired consistency is achieved.

Pour contents of the blender into a tall glass.

Serve immediately and enjoy!

Nutrition:

Calories per **serving:** 497

Protein: 28g

Carbs: 62g

Fat: 17g

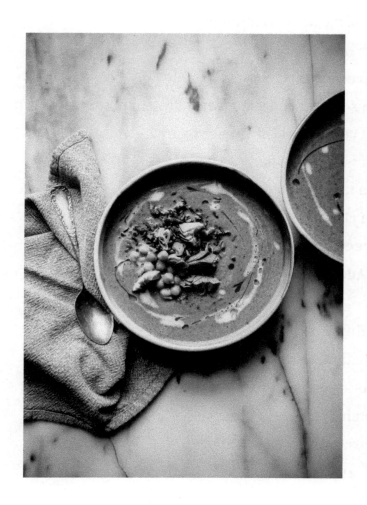

Chocolate Peanut Delight

Preparation time: 10 minutes

Cooking time: 0 minutes

Servings: 1

Ingredients:

  1 scoop of chocolate whey Protein powder

  1 cup of low-Fat Greek yogurt

  1 whole banana

  2 tablespoon of peanut butter

  1 cup of ice

Directions:

  Add all the **Ingredients:** to a blender and blend until
    smooth

  Enjoy

Nutrition:

Calories per **serving:** 656

Protein: 63g

Carbs: 55g

Fat: 21g

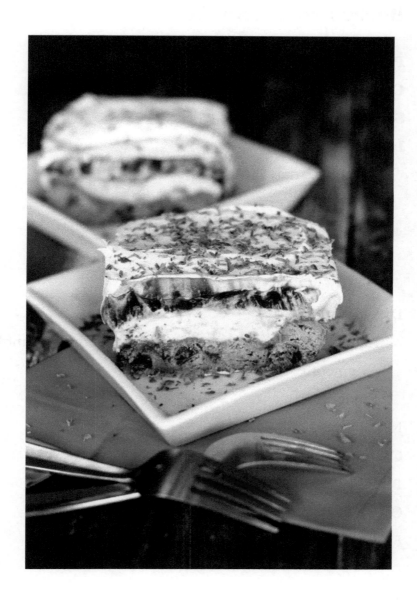

Berry Protein Shake

Preparation time: 10 minutes

Cooking time: 0 minutes

Servings: 1

Ingredients:

2 scoop of whey Protein powder

1 cup of blueberries

1 cup of blackberries

1 cup of raspberries

1 cup of water   1 cup of ice

Directions:

Add all the **Ingredients:** to a blender and blend until
smooth

Enjoy

Nutrition:

Calories per **serving:** 342

Protein: 38g

Carbs: 42g

Fat: 3g

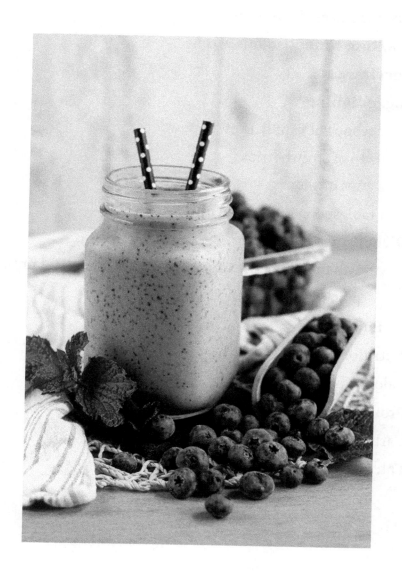

Fresh Strawberry Shake

Preparation time: 10 minutes

Cooking time: 0 minutes

Servings: 1

Ingredients:

   2 scoops of vanilla Protein powder

   1 cup of strawberries

   2 cups of water

   1 tablespoon of flaxseed oil

Directions:

   Add all the **Ingredients:** to a blender and blend until
      smooth

   Enjoy

Nutrition:

Calories per **serving:** 303

Protein: 35g

Carbs: 15g

Fat: 11g

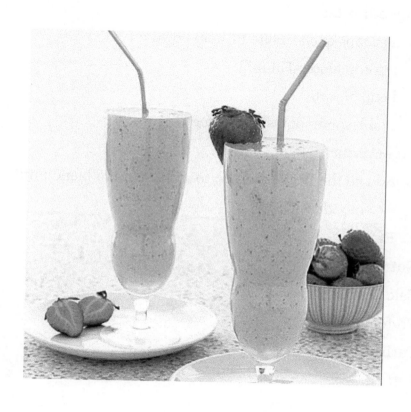

Choco Coffee Energy Shake

Preparation time: 10 minutes

Cooking time: 0 minutes

Servings: 1

Ingredients:

 2 scoops of chocolate Protein powder

 1/2 cup of low-Fat milk

 1 cup of water

 1 tablespoon of instant coffee

Directions:

 Add all the **Ingredients:** to a blender and blend until
 smooth

 Enjoy

Nutrition:

Calories per **serving:** 299

Protein: 42g

Carbs: 14g

Fat: 6g

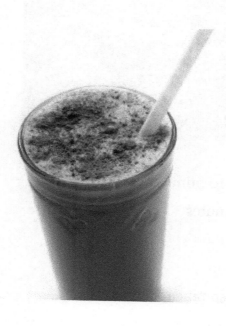

Lean and Mean Pineapple Shake

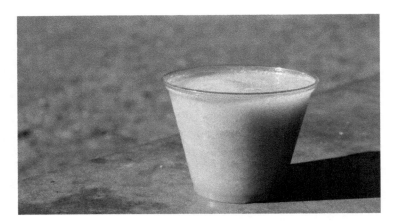

Preparation time: 10 minutes

Cooking time: 0 minutes

Servings: 1

Ingredients:

1 cup chopped fresh pineapple

4 strawberries

1 banana

1 tablespoon low-Fat Greek yogurt

1 scoop of vanilla Protein powder

1 cup of water

Directions:

Add all the **Ingredients:** to a blender and blend until smooth.

Enjoy

Nutrition

Calories per **serving:** 355

Protein: 23g

Carbs: 65g

Fat: 3g

Chopped Almond Smoothie

Preparation time: 10 minutes

Cooking time: 0 minutes

Servings: 1

Ingredients:

    1 1/2 cups water

    17 chopped almonds

    1/2 teaspoon coconut extract

    1 scoop chocolate Protein powder

Directions:

    Add all the **Ingredients:** to a blender and blend until smooth

    Enjoy

Nutrition:

Calories per **serving:** 241

Protein: 24g

Carbs: 6g

Fat: 13g

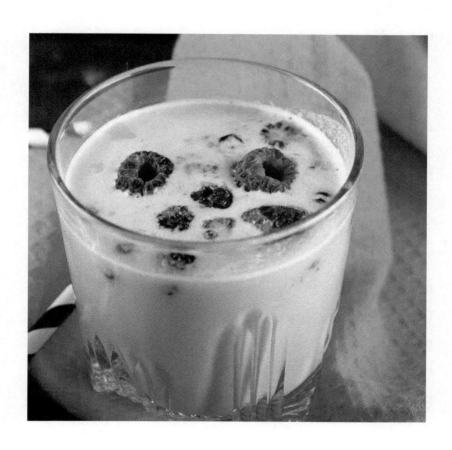

Vanilla Strawberry Surprise

Preparation time: 10 minutes

Cooking time: 0 minutes

Servings: 1

Ingredients:

2 scoops of vanilla Protein powder

1 cup of ice

1 banana

4 fresh or frozen strawberries

Directions:

Add all the **Ingredients:** to a blender and blend until smooth.

Enjoy

Nutrition:

Calories per **serving:** 329

Protein: 36g

Carbs: 42g

Fat: 2g

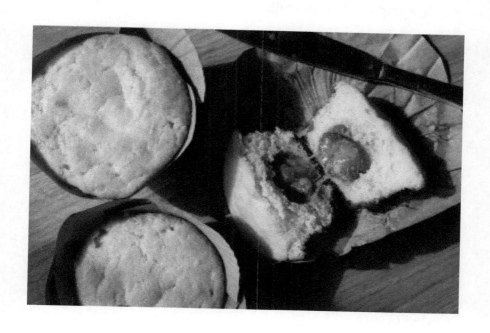

Breakfast Banana Shake

Preparation time: 10 minutes

Cooking time: 0 minutes

Servings: 1

Ingredients:

   3/4 cup of low-Fat milk

   1 banana

   1/4 pound of rolled oats

   2 scoops of vanilla whey Protein powder

Directions:

   Add all the **Ingredients:** to a blender and blend until
      smooth

   Enjoy

Nutrition:

Calories per **serving:** 566

Protein: 59g

Carbs: 69g

Fat: 6g

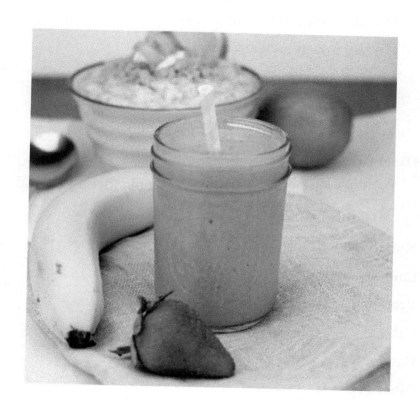

Berry Beetsicle Smoothie

Preparation time: 3 minutes

Servings: 1

Ingredients:

- 1/2 cup peeled and diced beets
- 1/2 cup frozen raspberries
- 1 frozen banana
- 1 tablespoon maple syrup
- 1 cup unsweetened soy or almond milk

Directions:

Combine all the **Ingredients:** in a blender and blend until smooth.

Nutrition:

Calories: 130,

Protein 9 g,

Fat 3 g,

Carbs 28 g,

Fiber 11 g

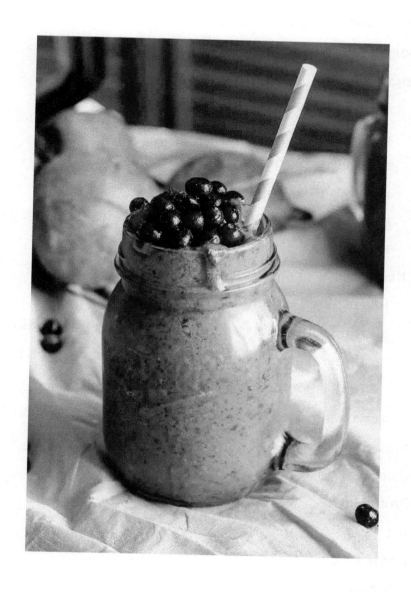

Green Breakfast Smoothie

Preparation time: 10 minutes

Servings: 2

Ingredients:

> 1/2 banana, sliced
>
> 2 cups spinach or other greens, such as kale
>
> 1 cup sliced berries of your choosing, fresh or frozen
>
> 1 orange, peeled and cut into segments
>
> 1 cup unsweetened non-dairy milk
>
> 1 cup ice

Directions:

> In a blender, combine all the **Ingredients:**.
>
> Starting with the blender on low speed, begin blending the smoothie, gradually increasing blender speed until smooth.
>
> Serve immediately.

Nutrition:

Calories: 100,

Protein 4 g,

Fat 3 g,

Carbs 20 g,

Fiber 10 g

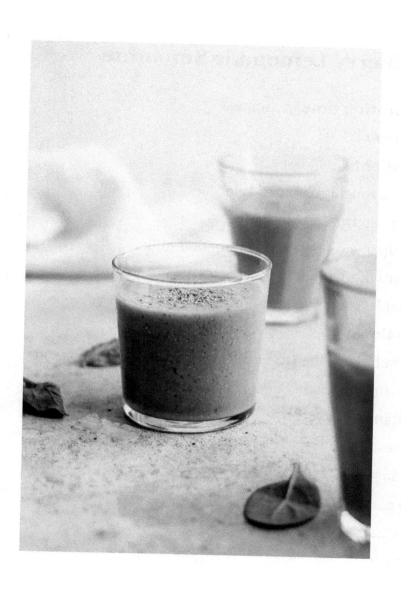

Blueberry Lemonade Smoothie

Preparation time: 5 minutes

Servings: 1

Ingredients:

    1 cup roughly chopped kale

    3/4 cup frozen blueberries

    1 cup unsweetened soy or almond milk

    Juice of 1 lemon

    1 tablespoon maple syrup

Directions:

Combine all the **Ingredients:** in a blender and blend until smooth. Serve immediately.

Nutrition:

Calories: 95,

Protein 5 g,

Fat 6 g,

Carbs 22 g,

Fiber 11 g

couponclippingcook.com

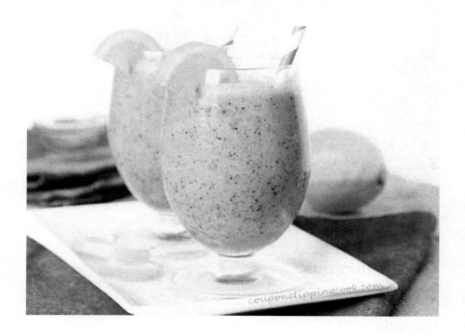

Berry Protein Smoothie

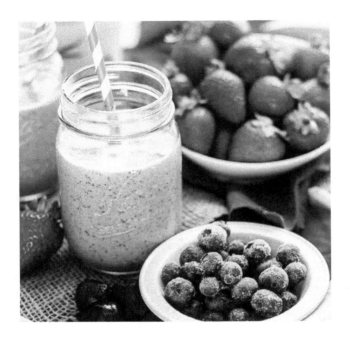

Preparation time: 5 minutes

Servings: 1

Ingredients:

    1 banana

    1 cup fresh or frozen berries

    3/4 cup water or nondairy milk, plus more as needed

    1 scoop plant-based Protein powder

    3 ounces silken tofu

    1/4 cup rolled oats, or ½ cup cooked quinoa

Additions

1 tablespoon ground flaxseed or chia seeds

1 handful fresh spinach or lettuce, or 1 chunk
cucumber

Coconut water to replace some of the liquid

Directions:

In a blender, combine the banana, berries, water, and
your choice of Protein. Add any addition
Ingredients: as desired. Purée until smooth and
creamy, about 50 seconds.

Add a bit more water if you like a thinner smoothie.

Nutrition:

Calories: 180, Protein 18 g, Fat 5 g, Carbs 30 g, Fiber 11 g

Chia Seed Smoothie

Preparation time: 5 minutes

Servings: 3

Ingredients:

1/4 teaspoon cinnamon

1 tablespoon ginger, fresh & grated

Pinch cardamom

1 tablespoon chia seeds

2 medjool dates, Pitted

1 cup alfalfa sprouts

1 cup water

1 banana

1/2 cup coconut milk, unsweetened

Directions:

Blend everything together until smooth. Serve
immediately.

Nutrition:

Calories: 210,

Protein 8 g,

Fat 9 g,

Carbs 25g,

Fiber 10 g

Mango Smoothie

Preparation time: 5 minutes

Servings: 3

Ingredients:

    1 carrot, peeled & chopped

    1 cup strawberries

    1 cup water

    1 cup peaches, chopped

    1 banana, frozen & sliced

    1 cup mango, chopped

Directions:

    Blend everything together until smooth. Serve immediately.

Nutrition:

Calories: 240,

Protein 5 g,

Fat 3 g,

Carbs 70 g,

Fiber 13 g

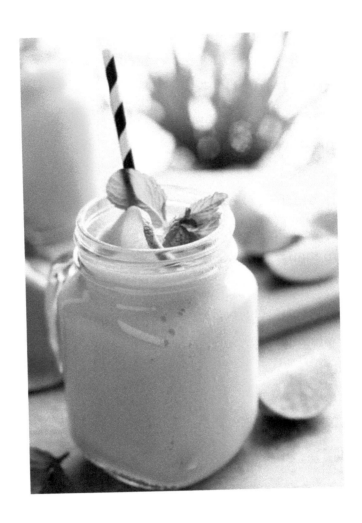

The Super Green

Preparation time: 10 minutes

Cooking time: 0 minutes

Servings: 1

Ingredients:

 1 tablespoon agave nectar

 1 bunch kale, spinach, Swiss chard or combination

 1 bunch cilantro

 2 cucumbers, chopped and peeled

 1 lime, peeled

 1 lemon, outer yellow peeled

 1 orange, peeled

 1/2 cup ice

Directions:

 Add all the listed **Ingredients:** to a blender

 Blend until you have a smooth and creamy texture

 Serve chilled and enjoy!

Nutrition:

Calories: 3180

Fat: 15g

Carbohydrates: 8g

Protein: 5g

The Wrinkle Fighter

Preparation time: 10 minutes

Cooking time: 0 minutes

Servings: 1

Ingredients:

 2 brazil nuts

 1 tablespoon flaxseeds

 1 orange, peeled and cut in half

 2 cups wild blueberries, frozen

 2 cups kale, roughly chopped

 1 1/2 cups cold coconut water

Directions:

 Add all the listed **Ingredients:** to a blender

 Blend until you have a smooth and creamy texture

 Serve chilled and enjoy!

Nutrition:

Calories: 180

Fat: 15g

Carbohydrates: 8g

Protein: 5g

The Anti-Aging Turmeric and Coconut Delight

Preparation time: 10 minutes

Cooking time: 0 minutes

Servings: 1

Ingredients:

- 1 tablespoon coconut oil
- 2 teaspoons chia seeds
- 1 teaspoon ground turmeric
- 1 banana, frozen
- 1/2 cup pineapple, diced
- 1 cup of coconut milk

Directions:

Add all the listed **Ingredients:** to a blender

Blend until you have a smooth and creamy texture

Serve chilled and enjoy!

Nutrition:

Calories: 430

Fat: 30g

Carbohydrates: 10g

Protein: 7g

The Anti-Aging Superfood Glass

Preparation time: 10 minutes

Cooking time: 0 minutes

Servings: 1

Ingredients:

   Water as needed

   1/2 cup unsweetened nut milk

   1-2 scoops vanilla Whey Protein

   1 tablespoon unrefined coconut oil

   1 tablespoon chia seeds

   1 tablespoon almond butter

   1/4 cup frozen blueberries

   1/2 stick frozen acai puree

Directions:

   Add all the listed **Ingredients:** to a blender

   Blend until you have a smooth and creamy texture

   Serve chilled and enjoy!

Nutrition:

Calories: 162

Fat: 14g

Carbohydrates: 10g

Protein: 3g

The Glass of Glowing Skin

Preparation time: 10 minutes

Cooking time: 0 minutes

Servings: 1

Ingredients:

   1/2 avocado, sliced

   2 cups kale

   1 cup mango, chopped

   1 cup pineapple, chopped

   2 frozen bananas, peeled and sliced

   1/2 cup of coconut water

   1 tablespoon flax

Directions:

   Add all the listed **Ingredients:** to a blender

   Blend until you have a smooth and creamy texture

   Serve chilled and enjoy!

Nutrition:

Calories: 430

Fat: 40g

Carbohydrates: 20g

Protein: 10g

The Feisty Goddess

Preparation time: 10 minutes

Cooking time: 0 minutes

Servings: 1

Ingredients:

   1 cup unsweetened almond milk

   2 tablespoons lemon juice

   2 tablespoons avocado, peeled and pit removed

   1 tablespoon sunflower seeds

   1/2 medium banana, ripe

   1 cup packed spinach

Directions:

   Add all the listed **Ingredients:** to a blender

   Blend until you have a smooth and creamy texture

   Serve chilled and enjoy!

Nutrition:

Calories: 401

Fat: 42g

Carbohydrates: 4g

Protein: 2g

The Breezy Blueberry

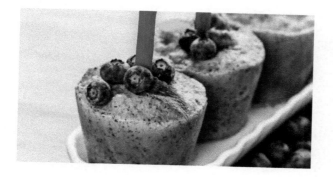

Preparation time: 10 minutes

Cooking time: 0 minutes

Servings: 1

Ingredients:

   Handful of mint

   1 teaspoon chia seeds

   1 tablespoon lemon juice

   1 cup of coconut water

   1 cup strawberries

   1 cup blueberries

Directions:

   Add all the listed **Ingredients:** to a blender

   Blend until you have a smooth and creamy texture

   Serve chilled and enjoy!

Nutrition:

Calories: 169

Fat: 13g

Carbohydrates: 11g

Protein: 6g

Powerful Kale and Carrot Glass

Preparation time: 10 minutes

Cooking time: 0 minutes

Servings: 1

Ingredients:

   1 cup of coconut water

   Lemon juice, 1 lemon

   1 green apple, core removed and chopped

   1 carrot, chopped

   1 cup kale

Directions:

   Add all the listed **Ingredients:** to a blender

   Blend until you have a smooth and creamy texture

   Serve chilled and enjoy!

Nutrition:

Calories: 116

Fat: 5g

Carbohydrates: 14g

Protein: 6g

Conclusion

In a nutshell, this cookbook offers you a world full of options to diversify your plant-based menu. People on this diet are usually seen struggling to choose between healthy food and flavor but, soon, they run out of the options. The selection of 250 recipes in this book is enough to adorn your dinner table with flavorsome, plant-based meals every day. Give each recipe a good read and try them out in the kitchen. You will experience tempting aromas and binding flavors every day.

The book is conceptualized with the idea of offering you a comprehensive view of a plant-based diet and how it can benefit the body. You may find the shift sudden, especially if you are a die-hard fan of non-vegetarian items. But you need not give up anything that you love. Eat everything in moderation.

The next step is to start experimenting with the different recipes in this book and see which ones are your favorites. Everyone has their favorite food, and you will surely find several of yours in this book. Start with breakfast and work your way through. You will be pleasantly surprised at how tasty a vegan meal really can be.

You will love reading this book, as it helps you to understand how revolutionary a plant-based diet can be. It will help you to make informed decisions as you move toward greater change for the greater good. What are you waiting for? Have you begun your journey on the path of the plant-based diet yet? If you haven't, do it now!

Now you have everything you need to get started making budget-friendly, healthy plant-based recipes. Just follow your basic shopping list and follow your meal plan to get started! It's easy to switch over to a plant-based diet if you have your meals planned out and temptation locked away. Don't forget to clean out your kitchen before starting, and you're sure to meet all your diet and health goals.

You need to plan if you are thinking about dieting. First, you can start slowly by just eating one meal a day, which is vegetarian and gradually increasing your number of vegetarian meals. Whenever you are struggling, ask your friend or family member to support you and keep you motivated. One important thing is also to be regularly accountable for not following the diet.

If dieting seems very important to you and you need to do it right, then it is recommended that you visit a professional such as a nutritionist or dietitian to discuss your dieting plan and optimizing it for the better.

No matter how much you want to lose weight, it is not advised that you decrease your calorie intake to an unhealthy level. Losing weight does not mean that you stop eating. It is done by carefully planning meals.

A plant-based diet is very easy once you get into it. At first, you will start to face a lot of difficulties, but if you start slowly, then you can face all the barriers and achieve your goal.

Swap out one unhealthy food item each week that you know is not helping you and put in its place one of the plant-based ingredients that you like. Then have some fun creating the many different recipes in this book. Find out what recipes you like the most so you can make them often and most of all; have some fun exploring all your recipe options.

Wish you good luck with the plant-based diet!

Lightning Source UK Ltd.
Milton Keynes UK
UKHW020657020421
381424UK00003B/28